Battling Pancreas Cancer
With
Nutrition

April Davis, MS, RD, ACSM CES
Kathy Beach, RN
Christopher M. Lee, MD

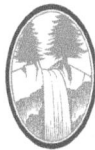

**PROVENIR
PUBLISHING**

Spokane, Washington

www.provenirpublishing.com

Battling Pancreas Cancer With Nutrition

This book includes text adapted from books in the *Living and Thriving with...* series published by Provenir Publishing with the editor's permission.

The authors, editors, and publisher have made every effort to provide accurate information. However, they are not responsible for errors, omissions, or for any outcomes related to the use of contents of this book and take no responsibility for the use of the products and procedures described. The editors, editorial board, sponsoring organization, and publisher do not assume responsibility for the statements expressed by the authors in their contributions. Treatments and side effects described in this book may not be applicable to all people; likewise, some people may require a different treatment than described herein due to individual circumstances. Drugs and medical devices are discussed, but may have limited availability controlled by the Food and Drug Administration (FDA) for use only in a research study or clinical trial. Research, clinical practice, and government relations often change the accepted standard in the field. When consideration is being given to use of any drug in a clinical setting, the health care provider or reader is responsible for determining the optimal treatment for an individual patient and is responsible for reviewing the most up-to-date recommendations on dose, precautions, and contra indications, and determining the appropriate usage for the product. This is especially important in the case of drugs that are new or seldom used.

Published by Provenir Publishing, LLC, P. O. Box 211, Greenacres, WA 99016-0211

Production Credits

Lead Editor: Christopher Lee

Production Director: Amy Harman

Art Director and Illustration: Micah Harman

Cover Design: Micah Harman

Printing History: April 2013, First Edition.

This book is dedicated to our patients and their families,
who inspire us every day in their cancer fight.

CONTENTS

Pancreatic cancer is a malignant neoplasm originating from abnormal cells arising in tissues forming the pancreas. The most common type of pancreatic cancer, which accounts for 95% of these tumors, is adenocarcinoma.

Pancreatic cancer is known to be an aggressive type of malignancy, and requires in many cases surgery, radiation, and chemotherapy treatments. Because of the aggressive nature of this diagnosis, treatment of pancreatic cancer requires a multidisciplinary team of physicians and care providers, including specialists in dietary needs and nutrition.

It is very common for patients with a cancer diagnosis to have many questions about nutrition and diet. In fact, this is one of the main ways that you (or your loved one) can aid yourself in the battle with cancer. The cancer can inhibit your body's ability to heal, decrease your energy, and decrease your immune system. By optimizing diet and nutrition, research has shown that outcomes of surgery, radiation, and chemotherapy are improved. This leads to improved cure rates, better cancer treatment outcomes, and greater ability for the body to heal and rebound from the effects of cancer therapy.

The goal of this text is to empower patients during their fight with cancer. By studying these practical approaches to health and nutrition, you can aid your cancer treatment team in your therapies. This is not meant to be a substitute for standard modern cancer treatments, but the goal is to provide you with further tools to fight cancer and improve your ability to heal from the cancer and the cancer treatments. Of course, this tool should be used in the context of your other treatments and we recommend that each patient discuss their individual health needs and objectives with their care providers.

PART ONE

Introduction

Nutrition plays a critical role in your overall health before and after treatment for pancreatic cancer. Pancreatic cancer affects the body's ability to digest and absorb vital nutrients from food. This can lead to nausea, taste changes, weight loss, fatigue, decreased appetite, abdominal pain, gas and bloating or diarrhea and constipation. Over time, these symptoms can put you at risk for malnutrition and loss of muscle mass.

Pancreatic cancer and its treatment can increase your body's need for calories and protein. You may have lost some weight leading up to your diagnosis and even more following surgery. Weight loss can contribute to fatigue, slower and longer recovery, and reduced quality of life. Therefore, it is important to equip yourself with best nutrition "tools" before and after surgery in order to maintain muscle stores and give yourself the best chance at having positive outcomes. This means choosing foods and supplements that can improve digestion and absorption, keep blood sugars stable, meet your body's nutritional needs, and support overall healing. There are even

more nutrition tools you can incorporate during chemotherapy and radiation to help decrease symptoms
and improve tolerance.

PART TWO

Nutrition Tools: Before & During Treatment

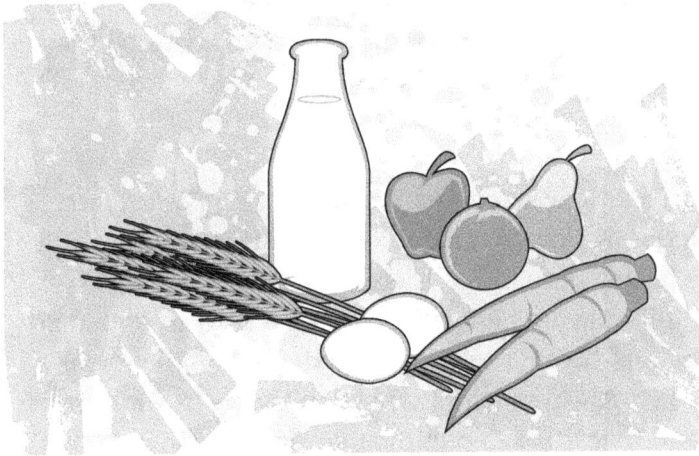

Focusing on nutrition can be the best thing that you can do for yourself during cancer therapy.

Before Treatment:

At the time of diagnosis, you may have experienced weight loss due to problems with eating, digestion, and/or fatigue. Difficulty digesting and absorbing nutrients from food can be one of the main side effects of pancreatic cancer. Depending on the location of the tumor within the pancreas and whether or not it has spread, treatment often involves surgery, chemotherapy, and radiation. Prior to having surgery, it is important to try to regain some of the weight and muscle tissue that was lost, if at all possible. The right amount and type of nutrition at this point can enhance your quality of life during and after treatment.

Many of the tips for improving nutrition status before treatment can also be used during and after to help maintain weight and health. Eating small meals or snacks increases the amount of nutrients that are digested and absorbed. Eating frequently assures that you are getting enough calories to meet your body's increased energy needs. It is also helpful to eat foods high in protein and low in fat. If you have a poor appetite, it may be beneficial to set an alarm to go off every 2 hours as your "cue" to eat.

You might have a hard time breaking down fatty foods, which can lead to discomfort in your gut and a feeling of fullness. Therefore, it is important to limit or avoid high fat foods, especially those that are animal-based, such as marbled meats and high fat dairy. Always include a protein source in your meals and snacks. Examples include: egg whites, lean cuts of poultry, fish, beans, low fat dairy, and whole soy foods. Eating these foods often can help you meet your protein needs and regain muscle tissue. Drinking enough fluids is another effective tool to feeling your best. Try to drink at least 8 cups per day, excluding caffeinated and alcoholic beverages. Vitamin D3 supplementation has been shown to improve immune health and mood, and cans be useful before, during, and after treatment (1, 2). You can also try nutritional supplement drinks, protein shakes, and other supplemental products. A Registered Dietitian can help you decided which supplement drinks are most appropriate for your situation. Typically, the products with at least 350 calories and 15 grams of protein in an 8 ounce container are going to be most effective. There is a sample 1-day menu at the end of this chapter that can help you visualize how to make these valuable changes.

NURSE'S NOTE:

Always consult your doctor before starting a new exercise program.

Nutrition Prescription Leading Up to Surgery:

• Eat small, frequent meals (every 1-1/2 to 2 hours, 6-8 times per day).

• Plan meals/snacks ahead of time.

• Set phone or watch to go off every 2 hours as a reminder to eat.

• Limit foods high in fat, especially animal-based fats.

• Include a high protein food in every meal or snack.

• Take a liquid multivitamin and consider additional vitamin D supplementation.

• Drink at least 8 cups of fluids per day, with at least 1/2 coming from a calorie-dense source, such as soups, smoothies, milkshakes, or supplement drinks.

Following Surgery:

Surgery for pancreatic cancer often involves removal of part of the pancreas, depending on where
the tumor is located. When the pancreas is function-
ing normally, it releases enzymes and insulin when
you eat a meal. Enzymes are proteins that help break
down nutrients. Insulin helps keep blood sugar stable
by bringing the sugars from your food into cells,
where it can be used for energy. Following surgery,
the amount of enzymes and insulin released by the
remaining pancreas may be less than what it was prior
to surgery. Pancreatic enzymes may be prescribed to
help your body absorb vital nutrients. If you experi-
ence stools that look oily, frothy, have a strong odor,
or float in the toilet water, you will likely benefit from
taking enzymes. It is important to talk to your doctor
or a Registered Dietitian about how much and what
type to take because it varies from person to person.

Insulin can be administered through a shot or
pump. For many patients with pancreatic cancer,
the need for supplemental insulin often depends on
whether or not your blood sugars were stable prior
to your diagnosis. If you have high blood sugar levels
(hyperglycemia) or diabetes, you will need to take insulin. You may need to be followed by an endocrinologist and a diabetic educator to assist with controlling
your blood sugar levels.

Other organs removed during surgery might include
your gallbladder and the first part of your small intestines, called the duodenum. The gallbladder stores
bile, which helps digest fat in meals. The duodenum is
where the majority of nutrients are absorbed by your

body. For all of these reasons, malabsorption, or the inability to absorb some nutrients, is a common side-effect of this type of surgery. At the same time, calorie and protein needs are higher when recovering from surgery. The great news is that your body is pretty amazing and can actually adapt to the loss of these organs over time.

While your body is learning to adapt, there are specific changes you can make to help absorb as many nutrients as possible and, therefore, lessen the amount of weight lost. Many of these tips are the same ones as before surgery, making it easier to transition. As previously mentioned, one additional tool is to take pancreatic enzymes before every meal or snack to help your body digest protein and fat. The amount and type of enzymes prescribed is based on your symptoms of malabsorption. Bile supplements can also be useful in helping to absorb the fat from your meals. Fat is a vital nutrient needed to meet your energy needs and absorb vitamins A, D, E, and K. Anything you can do to assist in digesting and absorbing protein and fat is particularly beneficial.

A specific type of fat that does not require enzymes for absorption is called MCT oil. Coconut oil contains a fair amount of MCT oil and is a terrific addition to your meals. You can use small amounts of coconut oil to cook with and/or add it to any soft foods to make them more calorie-dense. You can also purchase MCT oil in the form of caprylic acid in health food stores. A Registered Dietitian can work with you to decide how much caprylic acid to take during treatment.

NURSE'S NOTE:

Your nurse will weigh you at least weekly during treatment. This may occur more often if weight loss is a concern.

Omega-3 fatty acids are another type of healthy fat that you may want to consider supplementing. EPA and DHA are two specific types of omega-3 fatty acids that have been shown to be useful with pancreatic cancer. Research studies have found that EPA and DHA can slow tumor growth, decrease inflammation in the body, improve appetite, and lessen the amount of cancer-related weight loss (3-7). Talk to your doctor or a Registered Dietitian prior to beginning omega-3 fatty acid supplementation, especially if you are on a blood thinner such as Coumadin or warfarin.

Eating foods that are cooked over a long period of time (such as soups or meats/poultry cooked in a crockpot) can also improve absorption because the proteins in the food have already started to break down. Red meat is more difficult to digest than soft, tender fish and poultry. Again, remember that nutritional supplement drinks can give you an extra boost of calories, proteins, and vitamin and minerals in a small amount of volume.

NURSE'S NOTE:

Keep a complete list of medications in your wallet or purse. This list should include all natural supplements that you are taking as well.

If it is not possible to meet your calorie and protein needs through diet alone, you may need a feeding tube. Your doctor or a Registered Dietitian will let you know if this will be a useful option for you during treatment. A feeding tube is usually placed into the stomach wall and leads into your small intestines. A home health dietitian assists you in getting set up in your home with the appropriate type and amount of formula. They also teach you how to clean the tube and site and administer the formula. Getting nutrition this way can greatly improve absorption of nutrients because the fats and protein in the formula are already partially or fully broken down. To make this option less scary, keep the following points in mind: you are still encouraged to eat normally, as much as you can tolerate; no one will be able to tell you have a feeding tube when out in public; a feeding tube is not permanent and can be removed once you are able to meet your calorie, protein, and fluid needs through diet alone; and you will be closely followed by a healthcare team to make sure everything is working properly. It is much better to have a feeding tube placed, if needed, to help maintain your health than become severely malnourished and lessen your chance of having positive outcomes.

NURSE'S NOTE:

Ask your doctor or nurse about nutrition supplements.

Nutrition Prescription Following Surgery:

• Incorporate all of the tips from "Nutrition Prescription Leading Up to Surgery".

• Eat soft protein foods and cook poultry, fish and meats on low heat over a long period of time.

• Discuss the need for digestive enzymes, bile supplementation, and omega-3 fatty acid supplementation with your doctor or a Registered Dietitian.

• Supplement with MCT oil by adding caprylic acid and/or coconut oil to foods.

• Consider placement of feeding tube if unable to maintain weight.

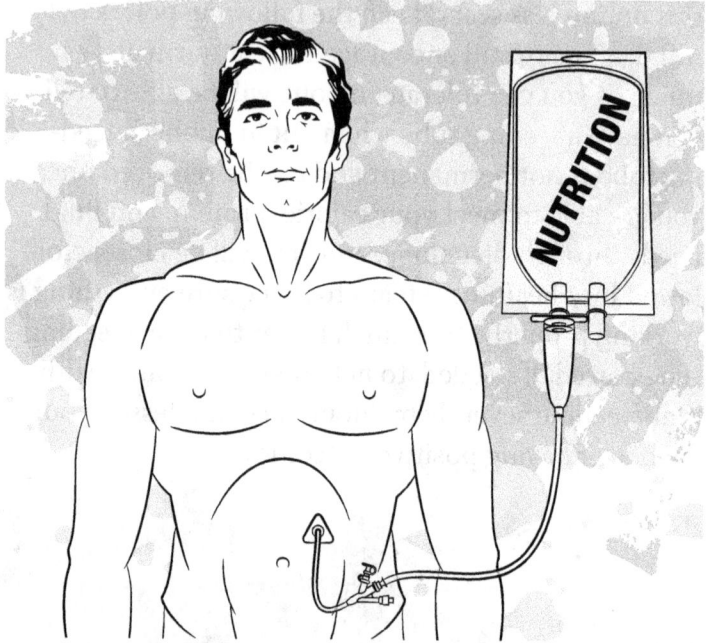

A feeding tube can become a "life-line" for you during radiation treatment if excessive weight loss is a problem.

During Chemotherapy & Radiation:

Many of the same nutrition tips that are useful before and after surgery apply during this phase, as well. Just like with surgery, your body needs extra calories and protein during chemotherapy and radiation. One big difference is that it is not recommended to take antioxidants in supplement form at this time. Some research indicates that supplemental antioxidants might interfere with chemotherapy and radiation (8). You should check your multivitamin to make sure it is not greater than 100% RDA or Daily Value for vitamins A, C, and E. These are strong antioxidants. You should also avoid taking any herbal supplements during chemotherapy and radiation. You can, however, continue supplementing vitamin D, enzymes, bile, omega-3 fatty acids, and a multivitamin (if it is not high in antioxidants). It is always encouraged to include whole food sources of antioxidants, such as blueberries and bell peppers, which do not interfere with treatment when eaten as part of a normal diet.

Chemotherapy and radiation can cause symptoms such as taste changes, mouth sores, nausea, and constipation or diarrhea. Each of these has its own nutrition-related toolkit that can be helpful in decreasing the degree of the symptom.

Tips for Taste Changes:

• Avoid your favorite foods 1 to 2 hours before and up to 3 hours after chemotherapy.

• Avoid eating where there are strong odors.

• Fresh fruits and vegetables usually taste better than frozen, canned, or cooked versions.

• Chilled or frozen foods may taste better than warm or hot foods. Use a baking soda/salt mouth rinse before eating (1 quart water, 3/4 tsp salt, 1 tsp baking soda).

• Use spices and seasoning to flavor foods that taste dull. Marinate meat, poultry, and fish for a more intense flavor.

• Use lime or lemon drops to flavor water. If you notice a metallic taste when eating, use plastic utensils and cook with glass containers, rather than aluminum ones.

NURSE'S NOTE:

If you use gum, mints, or hard candy to help with dry mouth, choose sugar free as sugar aids in the growth of yeast.

Tips for Mouth Sores:

• Use baking soda/salt mouth rinse often throughout the day.

• Coat your mouth with coconut oil three times per day, especially at bedtime.

• Avoid citrus juices and foods.

• Avoid spicy and hot-temperature foods and beverages.

• Avoid caffeinated and alcoholic beverages.

• Try warm, caffeine-free tea.

• Use a straw to bypass the mouth sores.

• Suck on sugar-free hard candy, frozen pieces of fruit, or ice chips.

Tips for Nausea:

• Take anti-nausea medication at the first signs of nausea.

• Sip on ginger or licorice root teas.

• Eat small, frequent meals and snacks.

• Avoid high fat and spicy foods.

• Stay adequately hydrated by sipping on fluids between meals.

NURSE'S NOTE:

If nausea is an issue, it may help to keep a food diary. This will help you decide which foods to eliminate during therapy to help alleviate side effects.

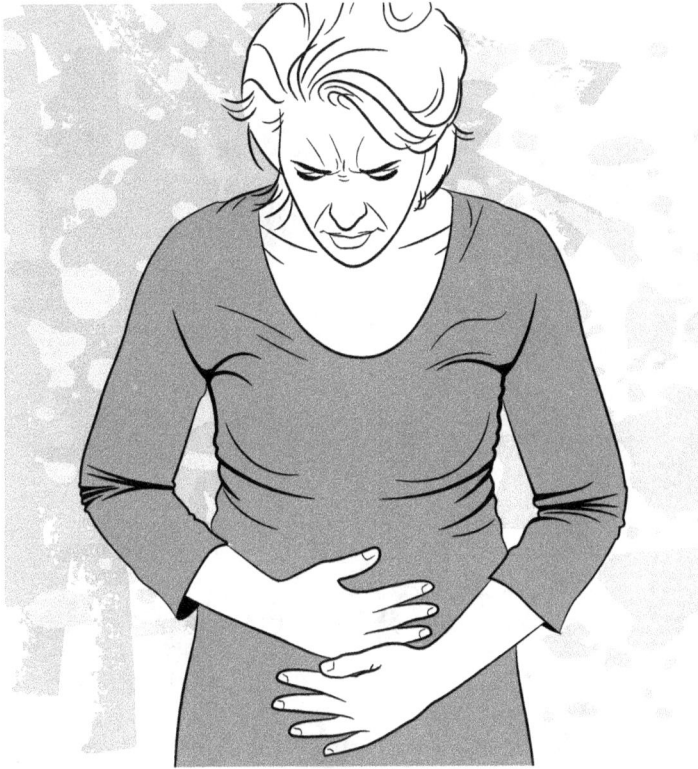

Let your providers know if you are experiencing nausea. With the many new medications available, nausea should not be a big issue for you.

Tips for Constipation:

• Eat foods high in insoluble fiber.

• Drink extra fluids – diluted apricot nectar can be especially helpful.

• Eat foods high in magnesium, such as roasted plantain chips, spinach, and beans.

• Replace your usual sweetener with molasses.

• Take Epsom salt baths.

• Move throughout the day, never sitting for more than 1 hour straight.

• Take a daily probiotics supplement.

Tips for Diarrhea:

• Follow the BRAT diet (bananas, rice, apple-sauce, and tea or toast).

• Include foods high in soluble fiber, such as coconut flakes, mango, and banana.

• Avoid foods high in insoluble fiber.

• Drink extra fluids, mainly broths, fennel tea, and electrolyte replacement drinks.

• Make rice congee.

• Take a daily probiotics supplement.

NURSE'S NOTE:

Remember caffeine can actually dehydrate you because it is a diuretic. You may want to cut down or eliminate caffeine completely during treatment.

The key to all of these tips is to make sure your food choices are appealing and well tolerated. Soft foods that are easy to chew, swallow, and digest are generally better tolerated than raw, crunchy, or tough foods. Choose foods such as egg whites, soups, Greek yogurt, hot cereals, noodles, soft poultry and fish, whole soy foods, and smoothies to help get you through chemotherapy and radiation.

PART THREE

Nutrition Tools: After Treatment

You may need to continue with the nutrition interventions adopted during treatment until all symptoms have subsided and your weight is back up. Once you are feeling closer to your "normal self", consider making some overall healthy lifestyle changes. The American Cancer Society's Guidelines on Diet, Nutrition, and Cancer Prevention recommend the following:

• Choose most of the foods you eat from plant sources.

• Eat five or more servings of fruits and vegetables each day.

• Eat other foods from plant sources, such as breads, cereals, grain products, rice, pasta, or beans several times a day.

- Limit your intake of high fat foods, particularly from animal sources.

- Choose foods low in fat.

- Limit consumption of meats, especially high-fat meats.

- Be physically active—achieve and maintain a healthy weight.

- Be at least moderately active for 30 minutes or more on most days of the week.

- Stay within your healthy weight range.

- Limit alcoholic beverages, if you drink at all.

Regaining muscle mass is a great starting point for exercise. Think about taking on a light resistance training program, such as "Workout to Go" from the National Institute for Health. You can download a free copy at: *www.nia.nih.gov/Go4Life*. Plan on doing one-third of the exercises each day, which will significantly improve your overall energy levels and quality of life. Once you feel strong enough, add on 15-30 minutes of low to moderate aerobic activity daily. This can include anything from briskly walking your dog around the neighborhood to cross country skiing to square dancing. Do whatever it is that brings you joy!

Sample 1-Day Menu

Set an alarm to remind you to eat every 2 hours during the daytime, with a goal of eating 8 times per day total. Amounts will vary slightly based on your individual estimated needs. Sip on fluids between meals, so that they do not interfere with being able to finish your meals/snacks.

Breakfast: 2 egg whites, mixed with 1/2 Tbsp MCT oil; 1 slice whole wheat toast with 1 Tbsp coconut oil and jelly spread on top.

30-60 minutes after breakfast: 3/4 cup herbal tea.

Snack: 1 cup (8 ounces) high protein nutritional supplement drink.

30-60 minutes after snack: 3/4 cup water.

Brunch: 1/2 cup tuna fish mixed with 1/2 Tbsp MCT oil and 1/2 Tbsp canola-based mayonnaise; 7-8 whole wheat crackers; 1/2 cup applesauce.

30-60 minutes after brunch: 3/4 cup herbal tea.

Snack: 1 skim mozzarella cheese stick; 1/2 cup canned pears or peaches in natural juice.

30-60 minutes after snack: 3/4 cup water
Late Lunch: 1 cup homemade chicken noodle soup.

30-60 minutes after late lunch: 3/4 cup herbal tea.

Snack: 1 cup (8 ounces) high protein nutritional supplement drink.

30-60 minutes after snack: 3/4 cup water
Dinner: 2-3 ounces tilapia baked in 1 cup plain Greek yogurt mixed with 1 ranch dressing seasoning packet; 1/2 cup cooked, soft green beans.

30-60 minutes after dinner: 3/4 cup herbal tea.

Snack: 3/4 cup (6 ounces) homemade high protein smoothie.

References

Trump DL, Deeb K, Johnson CS. *Vitamin D: Considerations in the continued development as an agent for cancer prevention and therapy.* Cancer J 2010; 16(1):1-9. Doi:10.1097/PPO.0b013e3181c51ee6.

Skinner HG, Michaud DS, Giovannucci E, et al. *Vitamin D intake and the risk for pancreatic cancer in two cohort studies.* Cancer Epidem Biomar 2006; 15(9):1688–1695.

Heller AR, Rossel T, Gottschlich B, et al. *Omega-3 fatty acids improve liver and pancreas function in postoperative cancer patients.* Int J Cancer 2004; 111:611-616.

Beck SA, Smith KL, Tisdale MJ. *Anticachectic and*

antitumor effect of eicosapentaenoic acid and its effect on protein turnover. Cancer Res 1991; 22:6089-6093.

Lai PB, Ross JA, Fearon KC, et al. *Cell cycle arrest and apoptosis in pancreatic cancer cells exposed to eicosapentaenoic acid in vitro.* Br J Cancer 1996; 74:1375-1383.

Merending N, Molinari R, Loppi B, et al. *Induction of apoptosis in human pancreatic cancer cells by docosahexaenoic acid.* Ann NY Acad Sci 2003; 1010:361-364.

Barber MD, Ross JA, Voss AC, et al. *The effect of an oral nutritional supplement enriched with fish oil on weight loss in patients with pancreatic cancer.* Br J Cancer 1999; 81(1):80-86.

Lawenda BD, Kelly KM, Ladas EJ, et al. *Should supplemental antioxidant administration be avoided during chemotherapy and radiation therapy?* J Natl Cancer Inst 2008; 100:773-783.

Journal

Common Cancer Terms

Adenocarcinoma: Cancer that originates from the glandular tissue of the body.

Adjuvant therapy: Treatment used in addition to the main form of therapy. It usually refers to treatment utilized after surgery. As an example, chemotherapy or radiation may be given after surgery to increase the chance of cure.

Angiogenesis: The process of forming new blood vessels. Some cancer therapies work by blocking angiogenesis, and this blocks nutrients from reaching cancer cells.

Antigen: A substance that triggers an immune response by the body. This immune response involves the body making antibodies.

Benign tumor: An abnormal growth that is not cancer and does not spread to other areas of the body.

Biopsy: The removal of a sample of tissue to detect whether cancer is present.

Brachytherapy: Internal radiation treatment given by placing radioactive seeds or pellets directly in the tumor or next to it.

Cancer: The process of cells growing out of control due to mutations in DNA.

Carcinoma: A malignant tumor (cancer) that starts in the lining layer of organs. The most frequent types are lung, breast, colon, and prostate.

Chemotherapy: Medicine usually given by an IV or in pill form to stop cancer cells from dividing and spreading.

Clinical Trials: Research studies that allow testing of new treatments or drugs and compare the outcomes to standard treatments. Before the new treatment is studied on patients, it is studied in the laboratory. The human studies are called clinical trials.

Computerized Axial Tomography: Otherwise known as a CT scan. This is a picture taken to evaluate the anatomy of the body in three dimensions.

Cytokine: A product of the immune system that may stimulate immunity and cause shrinkage of some cancers.

Deoxyribonucleic Acid: Otherwise known as DNA. The genetic blueprint found in the nucleus of the cell. The DNA holds information on cell growth, division, and function.

Enzyme: A protein that increases the rate of chemical reactions in living cells.

Excision: Surgical removal of a tumor.

Feeding tube: A flexible tube placed in the stomach through which nutrition can be given.

Gastro esophageal Reflux Disease (GERD): A condition in which stomach acid moves up into the esophagus and causes a burning sensation.

Genetic Testing: Tests performed to determine whether someone has certain genes which increase cancer risk.

Grade: A measurement of how abnormal a cell looks under a microscope. Cancers with more abnormal appearing cells (higher grade tumors) have the tendency to be faster growing and have a worse prognosis.

Hereditary Cancer Syndrome: Conditions that are associated with cancer development and can occur in family members because of a mutated gene.

Histology: A description of the cancer cells which can distinguish what part of the body the cells originated from.

Image-Guided Radiation Therapy: Also called IGRT. The process of obtaining frequent images during radiation therapy. These are used to position the radiation accurately.

Immunotherapy: Treatments that promote or support the body's immune system response to a disease such as cancer.

Intensity Modulated Radiation Therapy: Also known as IMRT. A complex type of radiation therapy where many beams are used. It spares surrounding normal tissues and treats the cancer with more precision.

Leukemia: Cancer of the blood or blood-forming organs. People with leukemia often have a noticeable increase in white blood cells (leukocytes).

Localized cancer: Cancer that has not spread to another part of the body.

Lymph nodes: Bean shaped structures that are the "filter" of the body. The fluid that passes through them is called lymph fluid and filters unwanted materials like cancer cells, bacteria, and viruses.

Malignant: A tumor that is cancer.

Metastasis: The spread of cancer cells to other parts of the body such as the lungs or bones.

Monoclonal Antibodies: Antibodies made in the lab to work as homing devices for cancer cells.

Mutation: A change in the DNA of a cell. Cancer is caused by mutations in the cell which lead to abnormal growth and function of the cell.

Neoadjuvant therapy: Systemic and/or radiation treatment given before surgery to shrink a tumor.

Osteoradionecrosis (Osteonecrosis): Damage to bone resulting from radiation doses.

Palliative treatment: Treatment that relieves symptoms, such as pain, but is not expected to cure the disease. Its main purpose is to improve the patient's quality of life.

Pathologist: A doctor trained to recognize tumor cells as benign or cancerous.

Positron Emission Tomography: Also known as a PET scan. This test is used to look at cell metabolism to recognize areas in the body where the cancer may be hiding.

Radiation therapy: Invisible high energy beams that can shrink or kill cancer cells.

Resection: Surgical removal of a tumor.

Recurrence: When cancer comes back after treatment.

Remission: Partial or complete disappearance of the signs and symptoms of cancer. This is not necessarily a cure.

Risk factors: Environmental and genetic factors that increase our chance of getting cancer.

Side effects: Unwanted effects of treatment such as hair loss, burns or rash on the skin, sore throat, etc.

Simulation: Mapping session where radiation is planned. If the doctor will be using a mask for your treatment, this is the time it will be custom fit for your face.

Staging: Tests that help to determine if the cancer has spread to lymph nodes or other organs.

Standard Therapy: The most commonly used and widely accepted form of treatment that has been tested and proven.

Targeted Therapy: Modern cancer treatments that attack the part of cancer cells that make them different from normal cells. Targeted agents tend to have different side effects than conventional chemotherapy drugs.

Tumor: A new growth of tissue which forms a lump on or inside the body that may or may not be cancerous.

About The Authors

April D. Davis, MS, RD, ACSM CES: As a combined Registered Dietitian and Clinical Exercise Specialist, April currently works as an oncology dietitian, supporting surgical, medical, and radiation oncologists and an endocrinologist. April helps cancer patients manage and prevent treatment side effects and provides tools to implement lasting diet and lifestyle changes for improved overall health. She has a Master of Science in Nutrition & Exercise Physiology and Bachelors of Science in Psychology, Biology, and Exercise Physiology & Metabolism. Prior to her current role, the dual credentials allowed April to work as a clinical pediatric dietitian, global nutrition and exercise consultant, university instructor, and cardiac and pulmonary rehabilitation exercise physiologist. She has also been involved in weight management workshops, health screenings, exercise prescription, and worksite wellness programs.

While working on her graduate degree, April received a fellowship in clinical nutrition and was elected outstanding student of the year by faculty members in the College of Pharmacy at Washington State University. April has given numerous lectures, seminars, and workshops on a wide range of topics at local, state, and regional professional conferences, including: Nutritional Issues Before, During, and After Cancer Treatment; Malnutrition Screening and Intervention for Patients with Cancer; Exercise Post Breast Cancer Treatment; Vitamin Diabetes?; Misinformation and Knowledge Gaps Related to Diabetes in Medical Rehabilitation Patients; Skeletal Muscle Plasticity with High Altitude Training; Effect of Aerobic Training on Cardiac Autonomic Regulation in Young Adults; Endothelial Progenitor Cells and Exercise in Children; Effects of Postoperative Exercise Therapy Following Lumbar Discectomy; and Ethnic Food Practices and Type 2 Diabetes in the United States.

Some of the past research April has focused on explored people's awareness of diabetes and how this information can be used as a guide for prevention and education programs. Information collected from this research was used to validate a diabetes assessment tool, identify strengths and weaknesses in domains of knowledge among patients at risk for or diagnosed with diabetes, encourage individuals at high diabetes risk to be more watchful for symptoms and pursue formal medical screening, and identify beliefs and attitudes surrounding misinformation. April has also developed a nutrition screening and intervention tool that has been implemented at an outpatient cancer treatment center.

April has traveled through the British Isles, India, Italy and the French Riviera as a consultant with an overseas travel organization to assess adherence to meal plans, portions, presentation, palatability, hydration status, activity level, and quality of foods served, as well as student satisfaction. She also writes monthly blogs to provide students and their parents' with tips on nutrition and physical activity pre and during travel, along with general advice on hydration, healthy travel snacks, and basic macronutrient education.

Volunteer work plays a vital role in April's professional and personal growth and she has served on two Boards of Directors for the Local and State Dietetic Associations. April also donates time facilitating nutritional workshops at churches, schools, and community organizations.

April is grateful to have had many unique opportunities in her career. It encourages her to spread her wings and delve into any and all possibilities with an open, creative mindset.

Kathy Beach, RN: Kathy graduated with her RN degree in 1993. She decided to get a degree in nursing after her mother was diagnosed with breast cancer. She spent sixteen years in hospital nursing where she worked on a wide range of units from Medical Oncology to Outpatient Surgery. For the past 4 years, she has focused her energy in oncology and radiation oncology with Cancer Care Northwest in Spokane, WA. She loves her work and finds the patients she cares for and their families to be extremely inspiring.

Christopher M. Lee, MD: Dr. Lee graduated cum laude in Biochemistry from Brigham Young University in 1997 which included a summer research fellowship at Harvard University and Brigham and Women's Hospital. He subsequently attended Saint Louis University School of Medicine where he received his M.D. with Distinction in Research degree. He completed four additional years of specialty training in Radiation Oncology at the Huntsman Cancer Hospital and University of Utah Medical Center during which he was given multiple national awards. Dr. Lee has actively pursued both basic science and clinical research throughout his career. He continues to be a proliferative author of scientific papers and regularly gives presentations on radiotherapy technique and the use of targeted radiation in the care of patients with head and neck (throat), brain, breast, gynecologic, and prostate malignancies.